a Mother's Blessing

Ayurvedic Wisdom for the Postpartum Mother

APARNA KHANOLKAR

Acknowledgement

Gratitude, appreciation and love for Lucinda Kinch for her beautiful cover art. Check out her inspiring works at www.lucindakinch.com

My sincere gratitude for all those who have come before me in cognizing this great wisdom and for sustaining it through the ages so we may benefit from it.

Deep appreciation and respect to my parents Pushpa and Anand Khanolkar for giving me the sacred gift of postpartum care after the birth of my children.

Deep bows to Benjamin and Anjali for their karmic nudges to transform me from girlhood to motherhood.

Hari Om

PREFACE

Aparna's clear, heartfelt and natural wisdom brings simplicity and common sense into the guidance of Ayurved for mothers as they bring their newborn through the veil, and onto planet Earth. It can't get any easier to gain such potent results. If you wish to prevent so many common problems, the core practices of successful postpartum traditions around the world are in your hands.

The three most potent things we can do to prevent problems after childbirth for mother and baby are in no particular order, 1) nurturing maternal rest, TLC, mothering the mother 2) warm oil massage daily for mother and baby, and 3) the unique dietary, oleation and herbal foods guidance for this sacred 6 - 8 week window.

Mother and baby are both so fragile after birth. We mothers have to choose and model self-care, and yes, there is time for it all.

Have a quiet intent and prayer for the best for your family, self-included - it is the best way to manifest support. Ma Nature wants the best for you all, it is evolutionary! In my 20 years as an AyurDoula and 15 years as trainer in this work, I still share in the delight in how quickly, often and profoundly we see improved quality of life for newborns, their mothers, and their family.

Yes, secrets to avoiding colic, lactation, hormone, mood imbalances and much more are embedded herein. If you need a little help, and of course that sometimes happens, AyurDoulas have more tips and tools to share with you, under the safe umbrella of your primary health practitioner, and in correct with an advanced Ayurvedic

3

practitioner if you wish.

The depth and breadth of a mother's blessing grows as the depth of her inner peace and integration in life grows. About both deep meditation and Ayurved, "Every mother should have this knowledge."... "Just get it to the people!" exhorted master teacher, Maharishi, Mahesh Yogi. Aparna is gifted at doing just this, and it is my honor to tell you, this book of simple measures is worth much more than its weight in gold.

So many blessings!

Ysha Oakes, LMT, CPAD

Dean and Founding Faculty
Sacred Window School

Table of Contents

For more information about Aparna's books and services, please visit:
www.themistressofspice.com/blog

"God could not be everywhere, so he created mothers." -- Jewish Proverb

Blessings upon you and your baby. Congratulations on choosing the most noble of paths. Being a mother is a gift to your baby and to the world. The grace, power and beauty of a mother is incomparable. A woman transforms into a mother through the qualities of devotion, love, patience, fortitude and commitment.

This book is for YOU. The knowledge and wisdom contained in this book is ancient but ageless, universal but timeless. Let it transport you to a realm where you are cherished, nurtured and held in Divine love.

What is Ayurveda?

The postpartum traditions of India, which are based on Ayurveda place equal emphasis on prenatal and postpartum care. It is clear that postpartum care for mothers is just as important as prenatal care. In India it is said that a woman has three rites of passage.

- Puberty
- Childbirth
- Menopause

Each rite of passage brings with it unique gifts and opportunities for bliss, joy and spiritual expansion. Ayurveda, the ancient science of healing from India is still alive and rich. It offers deep wisdom for all phases of a woman's life.

"Ayur" means longevity, "Veda" means science. The "Science of Longevity" has a special emphasis on mother-baby care. We use the wisdom of the Doshas to understand the physiological and emotional needs of the new mother.

Consciousness is the basis for all creation. Vedic science states that the goal of life is reaching pure consciousness. To experience and to be in a state of pure awareness and bliss is considered liberation. And Ayurveda supports this goal. The four Vedas: Rig, Sama, Yajur and Atharva have contributed great spiritual, psychological and lifestyle knowledge that is applicable to nearly all aspects of life. Vedic science clearly explains our connection and interdependence with the universe.

Saatva is the original quality of the cosmos and the mind. Cultivating saatva is done in various ways in Ayurveda. Forgiveness, meditation, right diet and life style, communing in Nature, being loving and practicing pranayama (breath work) are some of the ways to maintain a healthy intellect.

If one keeps the mind healthy with healthy habits and practices, one can achieve true bliss and happiness, which is one's divine birthright. The main spiritual focus of Ayurveda is returning to our original state of the soul or inner being and not allow external factors of life to draw us into our ego. This is especially important as you begin the journey of motherhood. Cultivating a harmonious, peaceful state of being is most essential for you and your baby.

Ayurveda is a most user-friendly system of healing. Unlike Western medicine where the patient expects or believes that the doctor can heal him by prescribing medication, Ayurveda empowers the patient to be fully involved in his own healing. Every aspect of healing is covered by Ayurveda be it rejuvenation, purification, strengthening or meditation.

Ayurvedic knowledge and its simple home practices are designed to educate and empower you to be fully involved in your own healing and well-being. This book offers you many such tools that you can implement in your home with minimal expense. What it requires is commitment on your part and a lot of self-love.

A most basic understanding of Ayurveda includes the study of doshas. Everything that is created in the Universe is composed of the five elements.

Fire

Water

Air

Space

Earth

These elements work in combinations and are known as Doshas and are responsible for functions in the body/mind.

Vata, a combination of Air and Space has the quality of movement. It is mobile, unpredictable, dry, cold and rough.

Pitta is composed on Fire and Water, which has the quality of heat, and is sharp and hot.

Kapha is a combination of Earth and Water and is steady, stable and heavy. A balance of these five elements results in health and happiness. When our doshas are balanced, our body function optimally, our mind is calm and clear. We are self-aware and our hearts sing and exude love.

The Doshas in the physiology:
Vata governs childbirth, menstruation, and excretion
Pitta governs digestion, metabolism
Kapha governs immunity, mucus secretions

Now that you know that Vata governs childbirth, it is important to pacify vata after birth. Vata and your digestive system are weakened and depleted from childbirth. Ayurveda emphasizes that we use simple ways to tone and strengthen it during the postpartum time.

In India, a new mother is given special care for 40 days as an investment in her health for the next 40 years. The years in between childbirth and menopause is a very special time of deep nurturance, caring for the body and mind. How to take care of yourself during that time determines your transition to menopause. An accumulation of imbalances in the doshas will impair not only your new mother experience; it will also affect the menopausal stage of life. The health of each stage of your life is dependent on the preceding one.

Follow the simple recommendations in this book and you will have a smooth journey during your postpartum time and you will set a solid foundation for ease during menopause and beyond.

Postpartum depression is almost unheard of in India and other old cultures because the women in the family and community take care of the new mother. A new mother is never left alone to care for herself, cook, do chores or care for her newborn

Studies in India show that new mothers who have nourishing and balancing food, emotional support, and daily oil massages have fewer incidences of postpartum depression, weight gain, emotional ups and downs. The journey of a new mother is a happy fulfilling one provided she receives the support and care from family and friends.

What is postpartum care?

Invest at least 40 days in your postpartum recovery. Have friends and family help you. Don't hesitate to ask for help and support. Yes, you are entitled to it. Mothers are creators. You have done such a big and important job of birthing your baby. Know that being a mother is the noblest of all paths. As families and communities we need to take care of our new mothers so they blossom into their new **"dharma"** or purpose with confidence, joy and courage. If your family is unaware of your need for support, ask for support or hire a doula.

Make these your top priorities:
- Nourishing food
- Silence for meditation
- Oil massage
- Rotation of friends and family to ensure you are free to rest

Before the baby arrives, plan with your spouse/partner as to who is taking over your responsibilities at home. This is not the time for guilt or martyrdom. Let the fast-paced energy of tasks be someone else's. Rest, bond with your baby and pay attention to the needs of your body and mind.

Meditation

Why meditate?

Meditation is the oldest technique of giving the mind deep rest and connecting to higher consciousness. When you meditate you feel refreshed and the nervous system is rejuvenated. Stresses are thrown out and you will experience a sense of calm and poise.

Meditating during your pregnancy is greatly beneficial to you and your baby. After the birth will help you recover faster from fatigue and exhaustion.

There are many forms of meditation. I practice "Transcendental Meditation," which is a mantra-based meditation practice. However, there are other techniques such as Vippasana meditation, open-eyed meditation technique, silent meditation which is without a mantra and affirmation-based meditation. Choose the one that appeals to you the most.

Meditate twice a day. Chant mantras while holding your baby or have your baby nearby. The healing vibrational are good for you and your baby. Within an hour after the birth of my daughter, I chanted mantras for her and played Vedic chants in the room. Friends came and chanted "Om" into my baby son's ears when he arrived home. Not only did these experiences create great memories, it also gave my children a sublime experience of the Divine soon after their arrival. Enjoy the deep silence of meditation as a gift from the Divine.

Mantra meditation is a wonderful practice of creating a vibration vortex that is healing and peaceful.

There are many mantras you can choose from. I've chosen for you a mantra that generates a feeling of peace, contentment for you and your baby.

If you are sleep deprived, a 15 minute meditation will give you the rest that you would get from a 2-3 hour nap. However, please don't substitute meditation for sleep. My meditation

practice gave me deep rest and a restored energy after the birth of my children. Whatever style of meditation you choose, know that your decision benefits you and your baby.

"Streem" (sometimes spelled as "strim") is the bija or seed sound for peace. "Stri" in Sanskrit means woman and so this is a Shakti energizing and peace generating mantra. It is stabilizing after birth and will help you regain your balance.

Feel free to practice this mantra before childbirth because it encourages a peaceful time during pregnancy.

OM STREEM DEVIYE NAMAHA

Chant this 108 times each day. If you are too exhausted then at least chant it 21 times. If you use a "japa mala" it will make counting easier. One round with the beads is 108. You can chant silently while counting the beads. Better still, chant audibly but softly. Let the sound vibration fall upon your baby.

Note: These mantras are not religious. They are seed sounds with powerful effects on your body and mind. You don't have to be practicing Hindu to chant mantras. The benefits of mantras are universal. The only requirement is sincere devotion to your practice.

Oil Massage

Practice the art of **"Abhyanga."** Heat oil, apply copious amounts to your body and let it soak in. Let the oil nourish your doshas and soften your skin and strengthen your bones and muscles. Take a hot shower afterwards and enjoy the deep bliss in the body.

Sesame oil is preferred as it is warming and thus balancing vata. Oil massages soothe the fatigued body and calm the nervous system. It is also known to tone the uterus and help detoxify the body. Special attention is paid to the back and abdominal region.

For the best quality oils, please visit:
www.banyanbotanicals.com

Instructions for Self-Massage

Abhyanga – The Art of Self-Massage

"The body of one who performs abhyanga regularly is not affected much even if subjected to accidental injuries, or strenuous work. By performing abhyanga daily, a person is endowed with pleasant touch, supple muscles and is strong, charming and is not affected by old age. "Charaka Samhita, a 5,000 years old Ayurvedic text.

Ideally, a trained Ayur-doula would come to you each day and massage you with hot oil. Abhyanga is the best way to reduce fatigue and pacify vata, aid in recovery from childbirth and give you feeling of deep relaxation. However, an Ayur-doula may not be available to you or costs maybe too high. In that case, practicing a self-abhyanga each day will be very beneficial as well. The health benefits of self-abhyanga are a gift to you for about a 15 minutes investment each day.

During your postpartum time, you must commit to a self-abhyanga each and every day. The optimal time for abhyanga is in the morning time. Try to avoid doing the self-massage after 5 p.m.

• Warm your dosha specific oil in a small pot on the stove or warm in a squirt bottle in a sink filled with hot water. Warm the oil to just above body temperature. Stand on a mat or an old towel, which can be washed.

• 5 tbsp. of oil or about 4 oz (depending on your height and weight) is a good amount of oil to cover the whole body. Pour a small amount of oil into a cupped hand, rub hands together carefully and apply to the scalp. Rub gently in small circles using your palms.

- Use circular motions on your face and over joints, long strokes over open areas and along limbs. Massaging the ears, palms of the hands and soles of the feet will stimulate nerve endings to help soothe the nervous system.

- Before moving off the towel or mat, wipe excess oil from the soles of your feet. Stand on a non-skid mat in the shower. Allow about 15 minutes for the oil to penetrate and absorb deeper.

- If you prefer not to wait, simply start your bath or shower, using water as hot as is comfortable and continue to massage your body. It is not advisable to put very hot water on the head or neck.

You don't have to massage your scalp every day. Do it at least three times a week because it soothes the mind.

You may feel hungry and fatigued after an Abhyanga. Eat a hot, nourishing meal and take a nap. When you wake up you will feel rejuvenated.

Please use the regular amount of shampoo for your hair, and apply it to your hair first, BEFORE you enter the shower. This will emulsify the oil and then you can add water and wash some more before rinsing. If you don't follow this procedure, you may end up shampooing your hair 3-4 times.

Caution: Oil residue can be dangerous in the dryer. Oil will wash out of fabric with hot water, a good detergent plus and some dishwashing detergent. Weather permitting; drying on a line outside would be best. Otherwise, dry the towels on low heat and check often to make sure it is safe. Remove the towels immediately upon drying to avoid spontaneous combustion.

Oils for Abhyanga

Generally unrefined organic sesame oil is best for the postpartum time. However, the following oils are good for the doshas.

Vata: Sesame oil

Pitta: Sunflower or Olive oil

Kapha: Mustard or sesame oil

To watch my self-massage video, please click on the link below

http://www.youtube.com/watch?v=718DbMBIy1E

Baby Massage

Massage your baby with warm oil each day after the cord falls off. This is an ancient Ayurvedic practice that you can incorporate easily into your daily life. The massage takes 10 minutes. The feeling of bonding and the pleasure of watching your little baby and knowing that you are nurturing her is a blissful experience. Before you begin your massage and bath, have everything ready nearby including your baby's clothing and diaper for after the massage. The entire experience should be a peaceful and luxurious one for your baby and you. Your baby's skin is delicate. Jewelry, rings and long and nails could hurt your baby accidentally. So keep your nails short and remove any jewelry before the massage.

- Warm 2 tablespoons of organic, unrefined sesame oil. Avoid essential oils and aromatherapy oils. Lay an old towel in a warm space in your room. Undress your baby. Place him on the towel face up.

- Take a small amount of oil in your hand and place it gently on the crown of the baby's head. Place the palm of your hand on the head for several moments.

- In India, it is said that the warm oil is nourishing to the fontanel region of the baby's head. If you massage, do so very gently. Your baby will love to stimulation to the scalp and head.

- Continue oiling your palms and fingers and use smooth, gentle but firm strokes to massage your baby.

Light circular movements on the chest and abdominal region, long strokes across the shoulders, downward movement on the arms and legs and upward movements on the back are deeply nourishing to your baby.

- When you finish massaging the front body, gently and carefully turn the baby over on to his belly and oil the scalp again. Move on to the neck and back using long strokes. Use more warm oil and massage the back using long strokes. Use the same technique for the legs. End with a gentle massage on the feet and toes of your baby.

- Singing and loving talk during the massage will keep your baby engaged and happy. Eye contact with the baby ensures him of your undivided attention.

When my mother massaged my newborns she sang to them, lovingly recited rhyming songs and spoke sweetly to them. They cooed along with her and received her love happily.

- Wrap the baby in a clean and warm towel after the massage and cuddle him before his bath.

Massaging the baby after a feeding is not recommended. If your baby develops a cold or fever, do not massage till he is fully recovered. In India, babies are massaged daily for an entire year. Daily oil massage will aid in digestion, immunity, strength and better sleep. You can massage your baby for years and when he is about 8 or 9 years old, you can teach him to massage himself.

Sleep

In India, the saying goes, **"Sleep when the baby sleeps."** When you sleep, the body heals, the mind is rejuvenated and the nervous system de-stresses. Waking refreshed to bond with your baby is important for your relationship. Fatigue can cause a feeling of being depressed. So sleep as much as you can. You will recover faster from childbirth. The quality of sleep before midnight is better and gives you deeper rest. Be in bed by 8 or 9 p.m. that way when you wake up for nightly feeding you will have already slept for a few hours.

Family and community

In India and in other older cultures, new mothers spend much time in the company of other women family members. Their life experience and wisdom alleviates any anxiety or confusion in the mind of the new mother. Trust the wisdom of experienced mothers who reflect your own parenting philosophy. Seek out their support and advice. They will be happy to help.

In addition to proper nutrition, it is a known fact that many cultures do not leave a mother alone to care for herself and the new baby. New mothers need tremendous support and rest and help in caring for other babies. In most ancient cultures older women in the family care for the new mother.

Mothers are nurtured during pregnancy and after birth as well. It is a special time for care and pampering by women family members. The expectant or new mother becomes the central figure in a family. Doulas can provide the same care to new mothers. This idea might be unheard of in the West, where mothers begin doing household chores, go shopping and attend social events soon after birth. However, good rest is exactly what the mother needs. A well-rested mother will bring confidence and joy to her baby. The focus of postpartum care should be on the mother, the new baby and the growing relationship between them. All other activities can wait till you are stronger and recovered.

Ask your mother or friends to come and hold your baby while you eat and rest. Babies love being held and you must take care of your own needs. Don't neglect yourself for the sake of the household chores. Besides, your family and friends will be thrilled to have the opportunity to help you and to bond with your baby.

Pregnancy aggravates vata as it inhibits the flow or movement of energy that is characteristic of vata. Respiration can be difficult as the baby grows in the womb and digestion is slow. This along with childbirth can create many imbalances that need pacifying and rejuvenation for strength and good health. The process of birth weakens the delicate nature of vata. Often mothers experience that weakness with symptoms of constipation and slow sluggish digestion.

After the initial euphoria of birth, many new mothers experience anxiety, deep fatigue and worry. These are qualities of imbalanced vata. Lack of sleep can exacerbate these tendencies.

So, frequent napping, good food and oily massages all help pacify vata.

Food as Nourishment to Tone and Strengthen the Body + Mind

There is nothing more nourishing to a new mother than a hot, nutritious fresh meal prepared with love. So new mothers require foods that are vata pacifying and nourishing, unctuous, grounding and easy to digest.

Cold drinks, smoothies, ice, juices and frozen foods are never served to a mother. As you know now, Vata qualities are cold and dry. Since the goal is to balance vata dosha, it is important to not consume cold foods. Boiled milk and water are served warm or hot. Drink plenty of hot water in between meals to pacify vata and to have a gentle cleanse for your digestive tract.

Look through the recipe section of this book. It contains many delicious recipes that are easy to prepare. All of the spices used in these recipes are available at your local health food store or grocery store. Purchasing the spices in small quantities before birth and "stocking" it might help in having them on hand to use right after birth. The recipes in this book have been used for women of many generations to aid healing and to increase milk supply. Now they are yours to enjoy and will help you nourish and strengthen after birth.

Edible resins are used in India to aid recovery after birth. The acacia gum resin is used along with raisins, almonds and wheat cooked in ghee to normalize reproductive organs after birth. After the tenth day, the mother is served one of these "gum balls" early in the morning with a cup of boiled cow's milk.

Vegetables such as tender green beans, carrots, opo squash, and different types of greens, zucchini and beets are served to the new mother. Along with vata -pacifying spices, the new mother is served ghee (clarified butter), to nourish and rejuvenate the body. Butter is never given to the mother as it has a cold effect.

Sour foods such as yogurt and tomatoes are not served often either as they are said to cause digestive problems. Instead "sweet yogurt" is served once a day. Sweet yogurt is homemade and is fermented no more than just a few hours.

Favor spices such as cumin, black pepper, cinnamon, cardamom, turmeric, fenugreek, dill, saffron and sea salt and in smaller amounts coriander and cayenne.

It is ideal if the food is prepared in small quantities, which is sufficient for one or two meals. Food that is stale, leftover and frozen is not appropriate for new mothers. It will further weaken your digestive fire. It is preferable that the vegetables are fresh and organic.

Meals should be served piping hot and the mother should sit down and eat comfortably and peacefully. If the baby is fussy or needs to be held, the doula or family member can hold the baby while the mother eats her meal. This will help with assimilation and proper digestion, all of which enables quick recovery from birth.

The new mother's diet may be considered rich because of her intake of ghee, but she is neither overfed nor underfed. The wisdom behind this principle is that the body after birth is in healing mode and the digestive system should not be taxed with overeating or eating heavy foods.

Another important factor in building digestive power is to eat meals on time. Breakfast by 8 am, lunch between noon and 1 p.m. and dinner between 6 and 7p.m. Your digestive fire or **Agni** is strongest between noon and 1 p.m. and it is optimal to eat lunch at that time.

All the loving care and nutrition that is provided to a new mother is intended to strengthen her for life and help her recuperate from the exhaustion and hard work of pregnancy and childbirth.

The expectant mother goes to her parent's home during the last trimester or the mother comes and stays with her daughter to provide care for her. This is a time for deep bonding between the mother and daughter and new ways of relating to one another are created. If that is not realistic for you, consider spending time with wise women friends. Seek their blessings, wisdom and support as you embark on this journey into motherhood.

In India, birthing is a rite of passage and the woman gains deeper intuition, wisdom and confidence in her femininity. After the birth, the new mother is not allowed to undergo any stress as it aggravates vata. Stress is known to hamper healing and can reduce milk production.

New mothers require and deserve a great deal of support and nourishment to heal their bodies and to fulfill their motherly responsibilities.In India, it is said that **If The Mother Is Happy Then Her Baby Is Happy.** So every effort is made and great care is taken to ensure the mother's needs are met and that she is happy.

Her health and happiness is vital for the blossoming of the mother-baby relationship.

Breastfeeding

After your baby is born, breastfeeding is the perfect bonding activity. Besides providing the most perfect nourishment for your baby, it is also a time to nurture your relationship with your baby. To know that your body can create and sustain a baby and give you the strength and ability to birth the baby and then create the most perfect food for that baby is a magical and miraculous.

Nurse your baby every two to three hours. This allows the baby to digest the previous meal completely and will help avoid gas and digestive discomfort. Drain both breasts completely. Drink plenty of warm water and herbal teas throughout the day. Make sure your foods are not stimulating, as this will stimulate the baby as well. Too much hot spice, fried food, meats, cheese, excessive garlic, fried food and too much meat will all alter the quality of your milk. Choose simple, easy to digest foods that are nourishing and delicious. Nurse in a quiet, warm and comfortable place. Do not indulge in heavy conversation, during eating or in other distracting activities such as watching television. Focus on nursing and enjoy this very special time.

If you have any problems or concerns regarding breastfeeding and need support, please feel free to contact your local La Leche League office. They offer free support.

New Beginnings

Life is magical, mystical and mysterious. There is life and death and life again. Each day we are renewed and rejuvenated as long as we are connected with the Divine. Especially now, at this sacred and special time in your life where you are bound to realize that your life is changing course and your purpose is being re-defined, commune with the Divine each day. For in that blissful silence, you will find all the support you need for this magical time in your life.

I recall standing under the starlight on a hot summer night with my newborn son and my father feeling an immense sense of wonder, gratitude and deep vulnerability knowing that the threads of karma had now bound three generations of my family together. I questioned myself in silence

"Who am I now? A young woman had been transformed into a mother through her children." And wondering what this would bring to my life's journey.

Today, my children are almost 13 and 9. A beautiful son and daughter - close to Nature, close to their innocence and consciousness. I wrote this book originally in 2003 after my daughter's birth.. To revise it after almost 9 years is a sweet experience.

Enjoy this magical time with your baby. Feel pride and joy in the fact that your body can take care of the baby you have birthed. And know your heart is expanding in unimaginable ways. You are blessed and fortunate. May you walk this noble path with courage, lightness, laughter, patience and support.

FEEL THE SUPPORT OF THE DIVINE, ALWAYS.

TEAS AND MILK DRINKS

Almond Milk

This is a rejuvenating milk drink that is said to increase milk production. Almonds are not only nutritious they also soothe the nervous system. It is important to peel the almonds not only because it is easier to digest but also because it contains trace amounts of toxins. Soy milk is nutritious but is not a good substitute as it does not contain the same energetic properties as cow's milk. Ayurveda advocates the use of boiled cow's milk even if the milk is pasteurized.

Ingredients:

6 almonds

1 cup whole milk

A pinch of saffron

1 tsp. turbinado sugar

¼ tsp. cardamom powder

Preparation:

Soak the almonds in water for about 2 hours. Then peel them and grind to a fine paste in a blender with some water. In a small pan, bring the milk to a boil on medium heat. Add the almond paste, saffron, turbinado sugar and cardamom powder and stir well. Drink it warm around bedtime or as a snack in between meals.

My tip: Soak almonds in hot water if you are short of time. White sugar is known to be vata aggravating as it is has cool and drying properties. Turbinado sugar or maple syrup is a good substitute as it is heavier and is in a more natural and whole form.

Poppy Seed Milk Drink

This is a soothing drink served to the new mother either in the morning or at bedtime. Poppy seeds are vata pacifying and are soothing for the new mother. Nutmeg also soothes the nervous system and induces sleep, both of which are necessary for proper healing after birth. Use nutmeg in small quantities -- a sprinkle suffices.

Ingredients:

1 tbsp. white poppy seeds

½ tsp. ghee

1 ½ cups whole milk

A pinch of saffron

1 ½ tsp. turbinado sugar

¼ tsp. cardamom powder

A pinch of nutmeg

Preparation:

Fry the poppy seeds in ghee for about 5 minutes on medium low heat. Stir often to avoid burning. Grind it in a blender with some of the milk till is somewhat smooth. Place the milk, poppy seed paste, turbinado sugar, saffron and cardamom in a pan and bring to a boil on medium heat. The consistency will be like that of porridge. Just before serving, add a pinch of nutmeg and drink it warm.

My tip: A micro plane grater is best for grating nutmeg.

Fenugreek Tea

This is a bitter-tasting seed. But it is known to increase milk production in the new mother and also detoxifies the body after birth.

Ingredients:

1 tsp. fenugreek seeds

2 cups of water

Honey or turbinado sugar to taste

Preparation:

Place the seeds and water in a pan and bring it to a boil. Let the tea simmer for about 5-8 minutes. Strain and drink it warm with honey or turbinado sugar.

Cumin Tea

This spice is used to reduce water retention in the new mother.

Ingredients:

1 tsp. cumin seeds

2 cups of water

Honey or turbinado sugar to taste.

Preparation:

Place the cumin seeds and water in a pan and bring it to a boil. Let the tea simmer for about 5-8 minutes. Strain and drink it warm with honey or turbinado sugar.

Fennel Tea

This is a delicious and soothing tea that aids digestion. It is also said to give a pleasant taste to breast milk.

Ingredients:

1 tsp. fennel seeds

2 cups of water

Honey or turbinado sugar to taste.

Preparation:

Place the fennel seeds and water in a pan and bring it to a boil. Let the tea simmer for about 5-8 minutes. Strain and drink it warm with honey or turbinado sugar. Alternately, fennel seeds can be chewed on after a meal.

Wild Celery Seed Tea

This is a strong spice with an intense flavor and should be used sparingly. New mothers are given this tea to pacify vata. However, excess use is said to reduce milk production, so use with caution. In northern India, this tea is given to new mothers for 40 days 2-3 times a day.

Ingredients:

1/2 tsp. wild celery seeds

2 cups of water

Honey or turbinado sugar to taste

Preparation:

Place the wild celery seeds and water in a pan and bring it to a boil. Let the tea simmer for about 5-8 minutes. Strain and drink it warm with honey or turbinado sugar. Alternately, fennel, cumin and wild celery seeds tea can be combined together to make tea.

SOUPS, MAIN DISHES,
AND SIDE DISHES

All recipes serve about 2-3

Homemade Ghee

Ingredients:

2 sticks unsalted butter Melt the butter on medium heat in a large pot. Continue to cook it till the milk solids separate and sink to the bottom. This will take about 8-10 minutes and you will see a golden liquid. There will be some foamy scum on the top. Once the ghee has cooled down, strain it into a glass jar and store at room temperature. Ghee does not need to be refrigerated because moisture that can turn it rancid has been cooked off.

Rice with Ghee and Black Pepper

At the beginning of lunch and dinner, serve the new mother two tablespoons of hot, freshly prepared rice along with one half teaspoon of ground black pepper, a little salt and a teaspoon of ghee. Black pepper is said to tone the uterus. The ghee will cut down the heat of the black pepper and provide much needed nourishment.

Postpartum Vegetable Soup

This is a warming, nourishing and easy to digest soup.

Ingredients:

2 tbsp. extra virgin olive oil or ghee

1 tsp. fenugreek seeds

¼ tsp. turmeric

2 cloves of garlic crushed

1 tsp. ginger grated

½ cup diced carrots

1/2 cup chopped green beans

½ cup chopped zucchini

½ cup chopped spinach

½ cup chopped fenugreek leaves

3 cups water

1 tsp. ground black pepper

1 tsp. salt

Juice of one half lime.

Preparation:

Heat the oil or ghee in a large pan. Add the fenugreek seeds and fry them on medium heat till they are golden brown, but not dark. Then add the garlic, turmeric and ginger and fry for about 30 seconds. Now add the vegetables and stir fry on high heat till they become bright colored. Add the water, black pepper and salt and bring to a boil. Turn the heat down to medium and cover and cook for about 14 minutes or till the vegetables are tender. Add the lime juice and serve it warm.

My tip: Fenugreek leaves are available at local Indian grocers in winter and in early spring. Discard the fibrous stems and use only the tops and leaves.

Postpartum Chicken Broth

Ingredients:

2 tsp. extra virgin olive oil

1 tsp. chopped garlic

1 tsp. ginger grated

6 or 8 organic chicken wings

4-5 cups water

½ cup finely chopped parsley

4 sticks of celery finely chopped

2 carrots finely chopped

1 ½ tsp. salt

1 ½ tsp. ground black pepper

Preparation:

Heat the oil in a medium-sized pot. Add the garlic and ginger and fry for about 30 seconds. Then add the chicken wings and turn up the heat to high. Stir fry for about 4 minutes and add the rest of the ingredients and bring to a boil. Cover and cook on medium heat for about 25 minutes. Remove the chicken wings and reserve it for some other use. Serve the broth hot to the new mother.

Semolina Pudding

This pudding is so delicious that anyone could eat it. But serve this nourishing and warm breakfast to the new mother every day at least during the 40 - day period. Wheat is said to absorb excess fluid in the body.

Ingredients:

4-6 tbsp. ghee

1 cup cream of wheat

3 cups of water

1/8 cup of slivered almonds

1/8 cup of raisins

½ tsp. cardamom powder

A pinch of saffron

¼ cup turbinado sugar

Preparation:

Place the 3 cups of water and turbinado sugar in a pot and allow it to come to a boil. Meanwhile, in a heavy bottomed pan, heat the ghee and stir in the cream of wheat. Roast on medium heat for about 8 minutes. Stir often to avoid burning. When the water comes to a boil, slowly add it to the cream of wheat and mix well. Add the almonds, raisins, cardamom powder and saffron and cook till the wheat absorbs all the water and thickens. Serve hot.

Dill Rice

Next to fenugreek, dill is one of the most commonly used herbs for new mothers. This dish is rich in fiber and is sure to please anyone who loves the unique taste of fresh dill greens. Dill is served frequently to new mothers as it is said to enhance milk production

.

Ingredients:

3 tbsp. extra virgin olive oil or ghee

1 tsp. cumin seeds

½ tsp. ginger grated

¼ tsp. turmeric

1 tsp. black pepper

1-2 bunches of fresh dill washed and chopped

1 ½ cups of Basmati rice

2 ¾ cups of water

1 tsp. salt

Preparation:

Heat the oil or ghee in a medium sized pot and add the cumin and ginger. Fry it for about 30 seconds and then add the turmeric, black pepper and dill and stir fry on medium high heat for about 4 minutes. Wash and drain the Basmati rice in three changes of water. Drain all the water and add it to the dill mixture. Stir fry on high heat for about 3 minutes and then add the water and salt and bring to a boil. Cover with a tight-fitting lid and turn the heat down to low. Let it cook for 16-18 minutes. Let it sit for about 5 minutes before serving.

Garlic Chutney

Garlic is used in many dishes that are especially prepared for the new mother. Garlic is said to maintain heat in the body, which is dispersed by the cold of vata and also detoxifies the body after birth. This chutney is potent and the mother should have about 1 tsp. a day for at least 40 days.

Ingredients:

½ cup peeled garlic

1 cup shredded coconut

4 tbsp. black peppercorns

½ tsp. coriander seeds

1 ¼ tsp. salt

The juice of 1 lime

4 tbsp. ghee

Preparation:

Heat 2 tbsp. of the ghee in a skillet on medium heat and add the garlic cloves. Fry it on medium heat for about 4 minutes. When it has cooled, grind the garlic along with the rest of the ingredients in a blender to a fine paste. Add a little water for ease in grinding. Heat the rest of the ghee and add the ground paste and fry on medium heat for about 12 minutes. This ensures that the garlic is cooked and the moisture has evaporated. This chutney can be served with hot rice or with some chapattis – Indian whole wheat bread.

Zucchini with Fenugreek

This side dish is perfect with chapattis – Indian flat bread.

Ingredients:

1 ½ tsp. extra virgin olive oil or ghee

1 tsp. cumin seeds

1 tsp. fenugreek seeds

½ tsp. Black pepper

¼ tsp. turmeric

¾ tsp. salt

1 tsp. coriander powder

2-3 medium zucchini cubed

1 small tomato coarsely chopped

Preparation:

Heat the oil or ghee on medium heat in a skillet. Add the cumin seeds and fenugreek and allow it to sizzle. After about 45 seconds, add the black pepper and turmeric and the cubed zucchini. Turn up the heat to high and stir fry for about 3 minutes. Then add the salt, coriander powder and tomato and mix well. Cover and cook for about 6 minutes or till the zucchini is tender. Serve warm.

Opo Squash

This side dish is easy to prepare and digest. Opo squash is a jade-colored vegetable that is about 12-15 inches long. It is available at the local Indian grocers, Asian grocers or specialty food stores.

Ingredients:

1 ½ tsp. extra virgin olive oil or ghee

1 tsp. cumin seeds

½ tsp. black pepper

¼ tsp. turmeric

¾ tsp. salt

1 tsp. coriander powder

1 medium opo squash peeled and cubed

Preparation:

Heat the oil or ghee on medium heat in a skillet. Add the cumin seeds and allow it to sizzle. After about 45 seconds, add the black pepper and turmeric and the cubed squash. Turn up the heat to high and stir fry for about 3 minutes. Then add the salt and coriander powder and mix well. Cover and cook for about 6 minutes or till the squash is tender. Serve warm.

Beets with Coconut

This is a savory side dish which is rich in iron and fiber.

Ingredients:

1 ½ tsp. extra virgin olive oil or ghee

½ tsp. black mustard seeds

½ tsp. black pepper

¾ tsp. salt

2 medium beets

1/8 cup shredded coconut

Preparation:

Cut off the tops of the beets. You can use beet greens in this dish or you can save it to prepare the vegetable soup recipe. If you purchased loose beets, cut off both ends of the beets and peel them and chop them coarsely.Heat the oil or ghee on medium heat in a skillet. Add the mustard seeds and place a lid on the skillet. After the mustard seeds pop, add the beets along with salt and pepper and stir fry for 3 minutes. Add about 4 tbsp. of water and cover and cook the beets for about 6 minutes or till they are tender. Add the shredded coconut and mix well. Serve warm.

Spinach Sabzi

Ingredients:

1 ½ tsp. extra virgin olive oil or ghee

2 cloves of garlic finely chopped

1 tsp. ginger grated

¼ tsp. turmeric

½ tsp. black pepper

¾ tsp. salt

1 bunch of spinach washed and coarsely chopped

Preparation:

Heat the oil or ghee on medium heat in a skillet. Add the chopped garlic and ginger and fry for about 45 seconds. Then add the turmeric and black pepper and spinach. Stir fry on high heat till the spinach wilts. Add the salt and cover and cook for about 6 minutes. Serve warm.

New Mother's Dal

This dish is made with moong dal and makes about 2 servings. Moong dal is easy to digest and the spices used in this dish help heal the new mother.

Ingredients:

¼ cup moong dal

2 tsp. extra virgin olive oil or ghee

1 tsp. cumin seeds

1 tsp. fenugreek seeds

¾ tsp. black pepper

¼ tsp. ginger grated

2 cloves of garlic

¼ tsp. turmeric

1 small Roma tomato chopped finely

1 tsp. salt

2 tbsp. finely chopped cilantro

Preparation:

Wash the moong dal in three changes of water. Cook with 3 cups of water in a crock pot or on the stove till the dal is cooked and is mushy. Heat the oil or ghee and add the cumin seeds, fenugreek seeds, black pepper, ginger, garlic and turmeric. Stir fry for about 45 seconds and then add the tomato. Fry the tomato for about 4 minutes and add the cooked dal, salt and chopped cilantro and bring to a boil. Simmer for about 5 minutes and serve hot with rice and beets or other vegetables.

My tip: If fresh fenugreek leaves are available to you, use the tops and leaves of one bunch. Add the leaves after stir frying the spices and allow it to cook for about 5 minutes before adding the tomato.

Pepper Chicken Curry

This is a spicy dish and is vata pacifying as it creates heat in the body.

Ingredients:

3 tbsp. extra virgin olive oil

1 cinnamon stick

1 tsp. cumin seeds

1 tsp. fennel seeds

1 tsp. poppy seeds

1 small onion thinly sliced

1 tsp. garlic chopped

1 tsp. ginger grated

1 ½ tsp. black pepper

¼ tsp. turmeric

2 boneless skinless organic chicken breasts

1 ½ tsp. salt

1 cup of water

4 tbsp. chopped cilantro

Preparation:

In a heavy bottomed pan, heat the oil and add the cinnamon, cumin, fennel, and poppy seeds to it. Allow it to become fragrant and then add the onion. Fry on medium heat for about 7 minutes or till the onions are soft. Then add the ginger and garlic and stir fry for about 30 seconds. Now add the chicken, black pepper, turmeric and salt and stir fry on high heat for 4 minutes. When the chicken browns, add water, cover and simmer for 15 minutes or till the chicken is cooked completely and the inside is not pink. Add the cilantro and serve with hot rice.

Moong Dal Khichari

This dish is an Ayurvedic classic for rejuvenating digestive fire. It is simple to prepare and is nourishing and vata pacifying for the new mother.

Ingredients:

¾ cup Basmati rice

¼ cup moong dal

1 tsp. salt

¼ tsp. turmeric

3 ½ cups of water

For seasoning:

2 tbsp. ghee

1 tsp. cumin seeds

2 cardamom pods

1 bay leaf

¾ tsp. black pepper

¼ tsp. turmeric

¼ tsp. ginger grated

Preparation:

Place the rice and moong dal in a pot and wash it in three changes of water. Drain completely. In a large pot, add the rice and moong dal along with the turmeric, salt and water and bring to a boil. Cover with a tight-fitting lid and cook on medium-low for about 18-20 minutes. When the rice and dal are almost cooked, heat the ghee and add the cumin seeds, cardamom and bay leaf and fry for about 45 seconds. Then add the black pepper, turmeric and ginger and fry for about 30 seconds. Add the spices to the cooked rice and moong dal and mix well. Serve immediately.

Fenugreek Raitha

This raitha is served as a side dish and is good for low digestive fire, which is common after birth.

Ingredients:

For sprouting:

3 tbsp. fenugreek seeds

1 cup of water

For seasoning:

1 tsp. extra virgin olive oil

½ tsp. mustard seeds

¼ tsp. turmeric

½ cup freshly prepared yogurt

½ tsp. salt

¼ tsp. black pepper

1 tsp. chopped cilantro

Preparation:

Soak the fenugreek seeds in water overnight. The next morning, drain the water and place the fenugreek seeds in a colander and cover it with a plate. It will have sprouted about 8-12 hours later. The sprouts should be about one half inch long. If the weather is cool, it might take longer for the seeds to sprout. Place the plate on the colander for a few more hours. Heat the oil in a small pan and the mustard seeds. Place a lid on the pan. After the mustard seeds pop, add the turmeric and the sprouts and stir fry for about 45 seconds. Add this to the rest of the ingredients and serve at room temperature.

Okra

This vegetable is soothing and strengthening to the
digestive system.

Ingredients:

1 tbsp. tender okra

2 tbsp. extra virgin olive oil

1 tsp. cumin seeds

2 small cloves of garlic chopped

¼ tsp. turmeric

½ tsp. black pepper

¾ tsp. salt

2 tsp. coriander powder

½ tsp. dry mango powder (amchoor) or ½ medium tomato chopped

Preparation:

Wash and dry the okra. Then trim the ends off and chop them into thin rounds. Heat the oil in a large skillet and add the cumin seeds. Allow it to sizzle for about 45 seconds. Then add the garlic, turmeric and black pepper. Stir for about 30 seconds. Then the okra and stir fry on high heat for about 4 minutes. Then turn the heat down and stir occasionally for about 12 minutes. Then add the salt, coriander powder and dry mango powder or tomato and continue to cook for another 5 minutes. Serve warm with chapattis or rice and dal.

My tip: The best way to make sure that okra is tender is to snap the end off. If it snaps readily, then it is tender. Some grocers allow customers to select individual okra in this way.

Asparagus with Spices

Asparagus is a vata-pacifying vegetable that can prepared for the new mother when it is in season.

Ingredients:

2 tbsp. extra virgin olive oil or ghee

1 tsp. fenugreek seeds

1 tsp. cumin seeds

¼ tsp. turmeric

1 tsp. ginger grated

2 cups chopped asparagus

1 tsp. salt

¼ cup water

2 tbsp. chopped fresh dill or 2 tbsp. chopped cilantro

Preparation:

Heat the oil in a skillet and add the fenugreek seeds and cumin. Allow it to sizzle for about 45 seconds. Then add the turmeric and ginger and fry for about 30 seconds. Now add the asparagus and stir fry on high heat for 2 minutes. Then add the water and place a tight-fitting lid on the skillet. Let the asparagus cook for about 3-4 minutes. Add the salt and dill or cilantro and cook for another 3 minutes and serve warm.

Fresh Yogurt

Ingredients:

1 cup whole organic milk

1/4 tsp plain organic yogurt

Preparation:

Boil milk for 5 to 10 minutes. Let the milk cool to 104 degrees Fahrenheit. Place the milk in a yogurt maker (or thermos etc.). Add yogurt starter (ordinary commercial yogurt is the simplest): 1/4 teaspoon in 1 cup milk; mix and leave the yogurt undisturbed for 5 - 7 hours. Unplug yogurt maker or other device. Leave the yogurt at room temperature until it is eaten at lunch. Do not refrigerate, as this makes the yogurt less wholesome.

Proper yogurt is:

a. Freshly prepared, which means started the evening before or the morning of the day of consumption.

b. Not yet very sour.

c. Well formed, i.e. of a semi-solid consistency which easily breaks up or which can be cut or "sliced".

Improper yogurt is:

a. Not well formed, which can mean:

- *Immature* and therefore slimy liquid, etc., due to the temperature being too low or the processing time being too short.

- *Sticky and thick* (a mass of porridge type consistency), due to the processing time being too long and/or the temperature being too low.

b. Distinctly sour, due to processing time being too long and/or temperature being too high.

c. Bitter in taste due to storage, much too long processing time, or a bad yogurt culture.

Lassi:

Mix 1 part yogurt with 3, 4, or 5 parts water according to preference. More water makes the lassi lighter to digest. Blend well.

Digestive Lassi:

Mix ½ cup yogurt, 2 cups room temperature water, ¼ tsp ground cumin, ¼ tsp salt in blender for 1-2 minutes. Skim foam off top. Makes enough for two large glasses.

Sweet Lassi:

Mix ½ cup yogurt, 2 cups room temperature water, ½ tsp Turbinado sugar, 4 drops rose water, ¼ tsp cardamom in blender for 1-2 minutes. Skim foam off top. Makes enough for two large glasses.

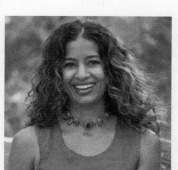

As a mother of a 13 year old and a 9 year old, I feel tremendous satisfaction in knowing that the postpartum care and love I received from my family has greatly contributed to my success as a mother. It is the greatest gift to a new mother. After the birth of my son, I became a postpartum doula myself and have served many mothers and babies. It pleases me to know that I have brought the ancient but universal traditions of India to the U.S.

I am a teacher at heart. I have taught hundreds of cooking classes, workshops on Ayurveda, have led retreats and have authored three books. A former chef of the Chopra Center for Well-Being in San Diego, I currently work as private chef for two families. I was also the Culinary Consultant to resort chefs across the US and Europe for Chopra Center programs in 2008-2009. These days much of my time is dedicated to creating and facilitating workshops for "Grace Power and Beauty" with my business partner Lisa Beck. We bring ancient Ayurvedic wisdom, music and dance to our modern lives so we can enjoy greater fulfillment, pleasure and meaning.

May this book serve you in the highest way.

Hari OM

On Facebook: The Mistress of Spice, Grace, Power and Beauty
www.themistressofspice.com
www.gracepowerandbeauty.blogspot.com

back cover photo credit: Tai Kerbs
www.photaigraphy.com
front cover art credit: Lucinda Kinch
www.lucindakinch.com

Made in the USA
Middletown, DE
09 October 2014